FIT, TRIM, SLIM

THE EASIEST AND MOST SUSTAINABLE WAY TO LOSE WEIGHT

BY RUXANDRA ANA MARIA DZUBAILA

I0412394

Table of Contents

Acknowledgements

Special thanks to ...

My mother, Adina Toma, without whom I would not be who I am today.

My lovely brother Mihai Dzubaila, for all his love, care and support.

Also to my soul sister Reema Vazirani who supported me unconditionally in the hardest times of my life, I would not be writing books now without her unconditional love.

And to my dear friend Richard Ewald, without whose unconditional help this book would not be here today. Richard is also a successful author and is helping writers at any stage of their career at his website: http://www.ePrompts.com

Introduction

One of the main stressors in my life was weight.

My first diet started when I was around 13, when my mother, worried about my weight, decided to take me to an endocrinologist. She wanted to check if I had any hormonal problems that had made me overweight and kept me that way. After the consultation, the doctor ruled I was healthy and I had no problem that would keep me from losing weight. He prescribed for me what was to be my first diet. It was my first diet, and the hardest one. Although my mother tried to make it as delicious as possible, suddenly having so many restrictions made me very unhappy. I remember I used to cry for a slice of bread. After few months on the diet I was fit and healthy, but it didn't last for long because in a couple of months I gained back all the weight I'd lost.

Seeing that and not wanting to go through the same diet, I started trying different diets from magazines.

This is what started my ongoing dieting. Even my cousin used to joke with me saying that, for all the time she's known me, I've been on a diet. That was true. I was for most of my life on a diet.

It was like an ongoing battle with extra weight.

I think I've tried hundreds of diets through my life, not to mention how many diet pills I have took effortlessly. It was like this until I learned about nutrition and exercise, at which point I started to see real results. But that was not enough because after a successful weight loss using just exercise and proper nutrition, I ended up gaining back the weight, and even more. Then I realized that weight loss is not only the result of diet and exercise. Weight loss is a much more complex process that involves a lot of psychology. I had no clue about it at that time, but I was determined to get answers and, as it says in the Bible, "seek and you shall find", this what I did. After years of trial and error, after years of research, I was finally starting to understand this complex issue of weight loss.

Weight loss is a mind game. Ruxandra's method.

I wrote this book because I see every day so many people going on crazy diets that put their health and their well-being at risk, in the same way that I once did.

This book is not a diet. It's a weight loss and psychological strategy to reach your desired weight and maintain it. It's not promising miracles. You have to *do* the work. To reach your desired goal of having a slim, fit, trim body you will need to make some changes, and these changes are sometimes psychological. However, don't worry. They are empowering, easy to make, and sustainable. But you have to *do* them. *You* must make these changes. *You* need to do the work.

What got you where you are right now is not going to get you to where you want to be. For things to get better, *you* have to get better. For things to change, *you* must change. This book is written very simply. I intentionally made it this way so you will understand it, and so it will be very easy to apply. If you follow exactly what is written in this book, I guarantee you will reach your desired weight goal. Achieving that will change your life. *You* will change your life. Because with weight loss comes a lot of good things, like higher self-esteem, confidence, joy, health, and an overall better feeling about yourself and your life. But you must *do* it. You must take action and make the changes needed in order to reach your goal. Already you took the first step, by buying this book. You are already a step closer to your goal. There is nothing to wait for. It's easy, practical, and you can do it.

FIRST PART

BODY

NUTRITION, EXERCISE AND SCIENCE

Weight Loss Is Mathematics

This is a very simple principle. How many calories[1] in, how many calories out? Deficit or surplus? This is what weight loss or weight gain is.

Your body burns a certain amount of calories per day, just to function. These calories are actually energy. For your heart to beat, for all your organs to function properly, they need energy, and this energy is usually taken from the food you consume. Now each person's basic energy consumption per day, without doing anything, is different. It depends on weight, age, sex, and height. Also, men burn more calories per day than women.

This is called Basal Metabolic Rate (BMR). Now feel free to go to the Internet, and calculate your BMR. Here is a link where you can do that:

http://www.thecalculatorsite.com/health/bmr-calculator.php

I repeat, this is what your body burns while resting in a normal environment, without the digestive process, when you have an empty stomach.

On top of this BMR, your body burns more calories during the day, while you are eating, drinking, walking, reading etc. Whatever you do, your body burns calories. And the amount of calories you burn depends on the effort your body requires. At the end of the day, the total calories you've burned equal your BMR calories plus the calories from activities. The more activities you do, the more calories you burn.

Now, let's look at an example. Let's say you hit the gym and burn 400 calories in an hour doing cardio. Now the total of the day will be: your BMR + your workout calories burned + calories from any small activities you do = number of calories you burned in that day. I must mention that if you do cardio, in that day your BMR will be higher because your metabolism for the next 24 hours will be very high. But if you go to the gym and do weight training, your BMR will be higher for 48 hours because it needs to do extra work to help your muscles recover.

Let's recap, the total calories you burn per day is your BMR (which can be the basic amount of calories, or higher if you hit the gym) + the calories from the activities you do (gym, walking, reading, playing, etc.) = the total amount of calories burned per day.

Now you have the number of how many calories you burn per day. To lose weight, you need to create a deficit daily. For example, if you are a woman and burn 2200 calories total per day (BMR + exercise, etc.) and you want to lose weight, you need to create a deficit of at most 1000 calories per day. That means that you should eat about 1200 to 1400 calories per day, for a healthy weight loss.

Let's say you're a man and the total calories per

day that you burn are 2600 calories. From this amount, you create a deficit of 1000 calories. So, you need to eat between 1600 and 1800 calories per day.

Now the deficit, or the difference between what you eat and what you burn, should not be more than 1000 calories. Also, for ladies the calorie intake per day should not be less than 1200 calories, and for men 1400 calories. The reason is this. If you make the deficit higher than 1000 calories, or if you eat under 1200 calories for women or 1400 calories for men, your body is going to enter starvation mode. This means your body is going to burn muscles for energy instead of fat. And you don't want this to happen because: the more muscles you have, the higher your BMR is; the less muscles you have, the lower your BMR is.

This is what happens when you follow a crazy diet, eating almost nothing. The scale immediately shows how many kg (pounds) you've lost, but what you've lost is not fat. It's mostly muscle. Also, if the body enters starvation mode, your BMR is going to slow down, because it needs to make sure you survive. It will not release the fat, and then when you start eating more, it will add more fat, because the body believes you're not going to give it enough fuel in the future. That's why most people who lose weight quickly with miracle diets end up gaining the weight back just as fast. They also usually end up even more overweight than they were before.

So, don't let your body enter starvation mode.

Maximum 1000 calories deficit, and not a calorie more. And not less than 1200 calories for women and 1400 calories for men. You can make the deficit less, 500 calories, that's fine. You will still lose weight. It will take more time, but you will get there. So, better slow and sustainable than never.

[1] - A *calorie* in this book is a *food calorie*, which is equal to one kilocalorie (kcal).

Why Diets Don't Work Long Term

I have around me many people who, for all the time I've known them, have been on diets. I was one of them myself. There are great diets: dissociated diet, meat diet, protein diet, 13-day diet, soup diet … there are so, so many. All these diets promise to change metabolism and change the way you store fat, and they deliver just that. Except not in a positive way.

But let me tell you something. None of these diets would ever work if they were not calorie restricted. For example, one might tell you to eat meat all day. But how much meat can you eat? 100 grams (3.5 ounces) of chicken is at most 200 calories. If you only eat this all day, after 500 grams (17.6 ounces) I'm sure you'll be fed up. Since it's protein, you won't feel hungry, but the calorie intake is at most 1000 calories. And even if you don't do any exercise you still can create a deficit of at least of 700 calories. If you have this deficit, of course you will lose weight. You're happy. The diet works. Then you tell everyone to go on it, and other people follow. They all say the same thing. The diet works.

Now, I must admit the diet really does work. In fact, if you follow any diet that has low calorie intake per day, of course it will work. But for how long, and with what price?

In the last few years, I've been telling my friends and family to count calories instead of going on crazy diets. During that time, my weight loss was slow and sustainable. For them, they lost weight, gained more back, lost it again, and then gained even more back. This is what happens on any diet.

Because, diets are not sustainable. Ok, let's say you're highly ambitious and for two or three months you're on a diet. You eat only soup or proteins, but all the time you're dying to eat chocolate. Three months later you've reached your goal. Now what? What do you eat? You're slim, so you don't need to keep doing the diet anymore. But you have strong cravings for chocolate and other delicious foods. You've ignored and suppressed your desires for such a long time. It occurs to you that you can now eat whatever you desire for one day. It's not going to affect you. The next day you will resume the diet. Wow, you felt amazing while eating all those delicious foods. The next day you are strong. You stick to the diet. The third day you might go out with friends. Now, because you held yourself back for so long, when you meet them and look at them eating all these delicious foods, in your mind you say to yourself: I can eat that too, one day won't hurt. Little by little you return to your old habits, and in no time, the weight you struggled so much to take off is back. And the same cycle begins again. However, you won't have the motivation to lose weight again until your discomfort reaches its threshold, but this time your threshold is not the same as it was in the past. Now your discomfort threshold won't start until you have even more body fat than you did when you started the diet the first time.

Diets are a vicious cycle. They don't work long term. The only thing that works is a new lifestyle. Suppression doesn't work long term, because the more you suppress and resist your desires, the more you want them. And dieting is suppression.

Your Eating Plan

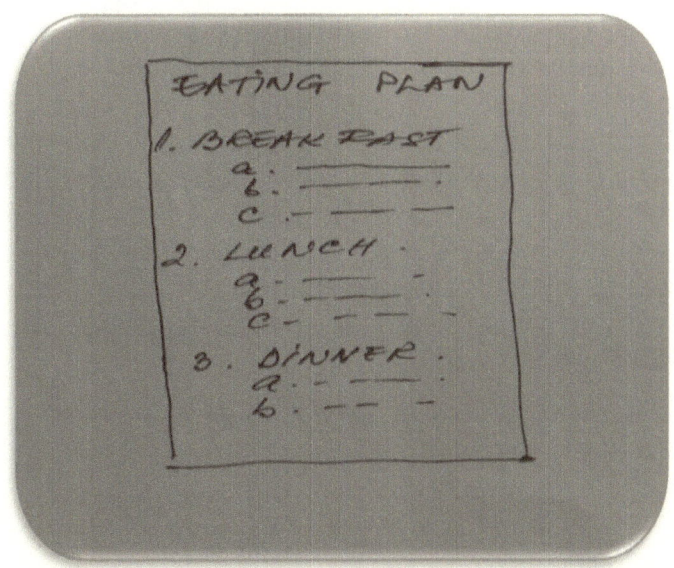

What will you eat from now on, so you can lose weight?

Here's an example you're going to love. If you want to eat chocolate all day and still lose weight, you can do it. That doesn't mean it's going to be healthy, but you can do it. For example, let's say you aim to eat 1200 calories per day and you like Twix or Bounty or Snickers. For each one of these bars, the normal size will have at most 300 calories. So, to make 1200 calories per day, you can eat 4 bars of chocolate per day. Isn't that fun! Eating Twix and losing weight. But it's not healthy to eat only this.

If you still want to eat chocolate, but also lose weight in a healthy way, you can. You could eat healthy foods for 900 calories all day, and have for dessert 300 calories Snickers chocolate. Isn't it fun? Losing weight while eating chocolate. And this works with any foods or cakes or whatever you like. You can still lose weight and eat your favorite foods. It is possible. If you are within your calories, you can eat anything. But know that it is important to eat healthy as well, because for healthy weight loss you need proper food. You need proteins, healthy carbohydrates, fibers. So, focus on eating healthy so you can get most of the nutrients you need.

I suggest this: 80% healthy eating and 20% whatever you like.

It's that simple. No suppression, cravings satisfied, balance, and eating healthy as well.

What does it mean to eat healthy?

It means that you need to eat the right foods in the right quantities. And here is what you need to eat.

Note: I am a vegetarian because I care about all animals and I can't eat them. For this purpose I cannot write a diet based on meat so I will be writing all vegetarian options, which you can feel free to combine with your eating choices. This is just to have knowledge of what you can eat. Thank you for your understanding.

To have a healthy diet you need to give your body the right nutrients. This means proteins, healthy carbohydrates, and healthy fats. In other words, this means fruits, vegetables, whole grains and cereals, proteins, dairy and oils.

Fruits: whenever possible, eat seasonal fresh fruits, along with those that are available all year. Some fruits are very high in calories, so please watch how many you are eating per day. Some of them they have very few calories, like berries and strawberries. Of these you can eat much more.

Vegetables: it is very important to eat vegetables, and the good part is that most of them are very low in calories, so you can fill yourself up with them.

Whole grains and cereals: on the first diet that I went on, the doctor recommended that I not eat bread. However, I don't agree with him now because healthy bread is good. There is still this myth that bread makes you fat, but this is totally wrong. Large quantities of bread make you fat. So, you can still enjoy eating bread, but this is what I suggest. Buy only whole grain bread, or any other bread that is not white, and make sure that it has no sugar or any other additives. Healthy bread will have a healthy flour, water, salt and maybe yeast. That's it. If it contains any other stuff don't buy it. Also, other things that are very healthy to eat will be oats, maize (corn), whole grain rice, wheat, quinoa etc.

Protein: is a much-needed nutrient for the proper functioning of the human body. According to the USA & Canadian guidelines, women aged between 19-70 need to consume 46 grams of protein per day and men between the same age should consume 56 grams of protein per day to avoid deficiency—or 0.8 grams of protein per kilogram of body weight (0.36 grams per pound). These guidelines are for sedentary people, but if you are an active person you would need much more than this.

Protein is very important not only for the proper functioning of your body, but also for your muscles. If your muscles don't get enough protein per day, you are going to start losing muscle mass. When this happens, your BMR will decrease because, as I said in a previous chapter, more muscle mass makes your BMR higher. That means more calories burned per day. But less muscles mass makes your BMR lower, resulting in fewer calories burned per day. Also, protein will keep you satiated for longer time, because it takes a longer time to digest protein than carbohydrates. The more protein you eat, the less hungry you will be. But don't go overboard with eating protein. Eat the right amount, and combine it with the other nutrients you need.

You can get protein from many things. Even fruits and vegetables have some protein. Dairy products. Whole grains and cereals have protein. Lentils have a lot of protein. There are many types of lentils with different nutritional values. All kinds of beans, peas, chickpeas, and nuts, like walnuts, peanuts, chestnuts, hazelnuts, macadamia, cashews, almonds, Brazil nuts, pecans, pine nuts etc.

On any product that you buy which has the nutritional guidelines, it will mention there how many grams of protein it has per 100 grams of product. With this you can estimate roughly how much protein you are eating per day.

Dairy products: there are many plant-based products that can give you the right nutrients you need, like plant-based milks from soy, from flaxseeds, from almonds. Not only they are delicious, but they are very healthy.

Oils: contrary to the popular belief that oil should be removed from a healthy diet, a healthy amount of oil per day is actually recommended. Although this should not be more than one spoon per day. Also, deep-fried foods are very unhealthy and toxic.

Oils to use: olive oil, coconut oil, grape seed oil, peanut oil, walnut oil, avocado oil, sesame oil.

But do not forget, even if is healthy, in the wrong quantities you are still going to put on weight. So, always check the quantity and calories before indulging in it.

Sugar

Although I still eat products with sugar, I try to keep it to a minimum. As I am a fan of chocolate and cakes, which all have sugar, I'm not going to completely quit those just because they have sugar. But on the side, I'm making sure that I don't take extra sugar unnecessarily.

I believe sugar is bad for health. Much research has confirmed that. Below I'm going to mention why. But before that, let me give you some advice. If you are a chocolate fan like I am, and you like chocolate from the market, then go for it. But be aware of the quantities, and also don't eat it every day. Indulging sometimes is okay, but at the same time, try to cut unnecessary sugar from your diet like I do. For example, I take coffee or teas plain with no sugar or sweetener at all. But if you don't like it this way and still want your drinks sweet, choose natural sweeteners like stevia. I've heard it's very good and healthy, and it doesn't have the damaging effect on your body that sugar has.

Also, check the products you usually buy from the market to see if they have sugar, and if they do, try not to buy those products. Look at other brands for alternatives. I found sugar in cans of beans, in cans of peas, in cans of corn, even in bread. In many products where sugar is not needed, they added it anyway so they can make it more appealing to your taste buds, so you come and buy that product again. Please don't choose those products. If you want to buy cans of beans or corn and you can't find any without sugar, go for the frozen ones instead. Most of them don't have sugar and are healthier than cans. Or go for the fresh ones. Bread, who needs sugar in their bread? No one. Sugar should not be there, but they still put it in because having sugar will create an addiction for that kind of bread. That's why many types of bread have sugar added. This is an unnecessary use of sugar that is damaging your body. Just choose the brands of foods and products that don't have sugar.

I was in India some time back, and I had no option for healthy bread. I have tried a sandwich with white bread. When I tasted the sandwich, believe me, I couldn't eat it. The bread was so sweet. It was full of sugar. And for what? We can eat bread without sugar. Bread is delicious enough without sugar. We don't need extra sugar in it. So please choose wisely. Please choose what you eat.

Having said that, your kids do need glucose while growing up for the development of the brain, but you don't need to give it to them from sugary products. You can make healthy alternatives that don't have sugar, and their bodies will take the glucose needed for healthy development of the brain. Don't take them to fast food. Don't give them junk food and sweets from the market. Give them healthy options. Because sugar is not healthy, and if they have a weight problem in childhood, they will most likely carry it with them into their adult lives. 1 kg (2.2 pounds) extra when they are small will be 10 kg (22 pounds) extra when are in their 20s. Choose wisely for yourself and for your children.

To illustrate for you how damaging sugar is, Dr. Nancy Appleton wrote on her website a list with 141 reasons showing how sugar ruins your health. Below is the list with some of the reasons mentioned. Please read them and spread the word:

Source www.nancyappleton.com
Reasons Sugar Ruins Your Health
By Nancy Appleton PhD & G.N. Jacobs

Sugar in soda, when consumed by children, results in the children drinking less milk.

Sugar can cause hyperactivity, anxiety, inability to concentrate and crankiness in children.

Sugar can produce a significant rise in triglycerides.

Sugar reduces the body's ability to defend against bacterial infection.

Sugar causes a decline in tissue elasticity and function – the more sugar you eat, the more elasticity and function you lose.

Sugar can lead to chromium deficiency.

Sugar can lead to ovarian cancer.

Sugar causes copper deficiency.

Sugar interferes with the body's absorption of calcium and magnesium.

Sugar can lead to an acidic digestive tract.

Sugar can cause a rapid rise of adrenaline levels in children.

Sugar can cause premature aging.

Sugar can lead to alcoholism.

Sugar can cause tooth decay.

Sugar can lead to obesity.

Sugar increases the risk of Crohn's disease and ulcerative colitis.

Sugar can cause gastric or duodenal ulcers.

Sugar can cause arthritis.

Sugar can cause learning disorders in school children.

Sugar assists the uncontrolled growth of Candida Albicans (yeast infections).

Sugar can cause heart disease.

Sugar can cause appendicitis.

Sugar can cause hemorrhoids.

Sugar can cause varicose veins.

Sugar can contribute to osteoporosis.

Sugar can lower the amount of Vitamin E in the blood.

Sugar can decrease the amount of growth hormones in the body.

Sugar can increase cholesterol.

Sugar can interfere with the absorption of protein.

Sugar causes food allergies.

Sugar can contribute to diabetes.

Sugar can cause toxemia during pregnancy.

Sugar can lead to eczema in children.

Sugar can cause cardiovascular disease.

Sugar can make the skin wrinkle.

Sugar can increase the size of the liver.

Sugar can increase the amount of liver fat.

Sugar can increase kidney size and produce pathological changes in the kidney.

Sugar can damage the pancreas.

Sugar can increase the body's fluid retention.

Sugar is the number one enemy of the bowel movement.

Sugar can cause headaches, including migraines.

Sugar plays a role in pancreatic cancer in women.

Sugar can adversely affect children's grades in school.

Sugar can cause depression.

Sugar increases the risk of gastric cancer.

Sugar can cause dyspepsia (indigestion).

Sugar can increase the risk of developing gout.

Sugar reduces learning capacity.

Sugar can contribute to Alzheimer's disease.

Sugar can cause hormonal imbalance

Sugar can lead to the formation of kidney stones.

Sugar can lead to biliary tract cancer.

Sugar slows food's travel time through the gastrointestinal tract.

Sugar is an addictive substance.

Sugar can be intoxicating, similar to alcohol.

Sugar can aggravate premenstrual syndrome (PMS).

Sugar can decrease emotional stability.

Sugar promotes excessive food intake in obese

Sugar can slow the ability of the adrenal glands to function.

Sugar is a risk factor for lung cancer.

Sugar increases the risk of polio.

Sugar can cause epileptic seizures.

Sugar can increase systolic blood pressure (pressure when the heart is contracting).

Sugar can induce cell death.

Sugar can increase the amount of food that you eat.

Sugar can cause antisocial behavior in juvenile delinquents.

Sugar can lead to prostate cancer.

Sugar dehydrates newborns.

Sugar can cause women to give birth to babies with low birth weight.

Sugar is associated with a worse outcome of schizophrenia.

Sugar can raise homocysteine levels in the bloodstream.

Sugar increases the risk of breast cancer.

Sugar is a risk factor in small intestine cancer.

Sugar can cause laryngeal cancer.

Sugar induces salt and water retention.

Sugar can contribute to mild memory loss.

Sugar water, when given to children shortly after birth, results in those children preferring sugar water to regular water throughout childhood.

Sugar causes constipation.

Sugar can cause brain decay in pre-diabetic and diabetic women.

Sugar can increase the risk of stomach cancer.

Sugar can cause metabolic syndrome.

Sugar can cause asthma.

Sugar can cause endometrial cancer.

Sugar can cause renal (kidney) cell cancer.

Sugar can cause liver tumors.

Sugar plays a role in the cause and the continuation of acne.

Sugar can ruin the sex life of both men and women by turning off the gene that controls the sex hormones.

Sugar can cause fatigue, moodiness, nervousness, and depression.

Sugar can make many essential nutrients less available to cells.

Sugar can increase uric acid in blood.

Sugar can lead to higher C-peptide concentrations.

Sugar causes inflammation.

Sugar can decrease testosterone production.

As mentioned above, you have so many reasons to reduce sugar from your diet as much as you can. If you cannot do it all at once, try with small steps that will lead to big ones. Little by little every day until your sugar intake will decrease.

Breakfast

"Breakfast is the most important meal of the day." Whoever said that was very right, and here's why.

Breakfast comes after so many hours of your body not getting any liquids or food. If you eat the last meal in the evening between 6 and 8 pm, and the next day let's say you wake up at 8, you have already gone a minimum of 12 hours, during which your body was practically starved. Of course, this is good to have all these hours without eating in order to get good sleep. Because your metabolism should not be focusing on digestion but rather on slowing down and letting you sleep. That's why it's not good to sleep with a full stomach, and it's important to have at least 2 to 3 hours since your last meal before you sleep.

Once you sleep, if you didn't eat right before you sleep (which, I'd like to stress again ... don't sleep just after eating), the metabolism slows down, but not completely. It slows down and focuses only on the proper functioning of your organs, like keeping your heart beating, blood flowing, brain functioning, etc.

When you wake up in the morning and once you are up, your metabolism starts to speed up. That's why you have energy when you wake up, even though you didn't drink or eat for so many hours. At least you should have enough energy. If you don't then you should check if your diet is healthy. If it's unhealthy, then no wonder you don't wake up with energy.

Now the next thing you must do to keep your energy up is to drink water. Your body already is dehydrated, since you didn't drink water for so many hours. If you fail to do so and you don't drink water, your metabolism will slow down, trying to function with what it has, and your energy levels will go down. After you drink water, within at most one hour you must have breakfast. If you don't have breakfast, and you choose to just grab a coffee and start your day, then your body, which is dehydrated and already starved, will enter to starvation mode.

As I explained in the chapter *Weight Loss Is Mathematics*, once the body is in starvation mode, the metabolism will slow down. It will start storing fat and taking energy from muscles, and next time you eat, you are going to gain fat.

There has been much research showing that people who don't eat breakfast are most likely to become obese.

Breakfast is not only a must for successful weight loss, but it's a must in any person's life for their wellbeing and healthy lifestyle.

So, having said that, choose wisely. Give your body what it needs. That means water and food, from the start of the day.

Don't skip breakfast!

Basic Exercise

It's good to do some form of exercise, and nowadays everything is available from the comfort of your home. If you don't like to hit the gym, and you don't have any medical conditions, YouTube has hundreds, thousands of workouts that you can do, for beginners to professional athletes. From yoga, to cardio dance workout, strength, whatever you like. It's available on YouTube for free, and you can do it from the comfort of your home. But if you don't like to do workouts at all, then go biking, go walking, take the stairs instead of the elevator, go to a disco and go dancing. Every day do something that speeds up your metabolism and makes you more energetic and alive.

If you decided to start exercising that's fabulous, because nutrition by itself is not enough to have that trim body. Although you can be slim by only focusing on nutrition, without exercise you will not be toned and trim.

Now there are many myths around exercise, and some of them I would like to share with you to debunk them.

Myth 1: Lifting weights will make you bulky and muscular like Arnold.

Well, it can make you more muscular, but not by chance. For the muscles to grow that big you must take supplements to encourage that growth, not to mention one really needs to lift incredible weights. And it will take years to reach that result.

Also, one cannot reach that result by chance, or just by lifting weights, because muscle growth is determined by the levels of the testosterone you have in your body.

Know that men's bodies produce much more testosterone than women's bodies. That's why, even if they don't lift weights, their muscles are usually bigger.

A man who is regularly lifting weights and eating healthy, and who is not taking any supplements for growth, will not have bulky muscles. He will have strong and well-defined muscles, but he will not have growth like someone who is training for a bodybuilding contest.

Also, for ladies there are a lot of misconceptions about lifting weights. I've heard that many ladies who go to gym just do cardio because they believe that lifting weights is going to make them have lots of muscles and make them masculine. This is a myth. Because women's bodies don't produce enough testosterone for the muscles to grow like men's.

For example, for many years I've lifted weights in the gym, but I don't have a muscular body. I have a more toned body.

There are many ladies at the gym who lift incredible amount of weights, and guess what, they are not muscular. They are slim, trim, thin, and toned. I repeat, if someone is very bulky and muscular and is lifting weights, it's almost always because of taking supplements for growth.

I would say, it is safe for women and men to go

and lift weights, and in fact it's a must in your exercise routine. Cardio alone is not enough for your body. Some strength workout is necessary, and this can be by lifting weights or doing body strength exercises.

Myth 2: If I go to gym, I can eat whatever I want. Wrong. Going to the gym is not going to guarantee the success of your weight loss. What you put on the plate is equally important as exercise. So do both.

When I started exercising many years back, I thought that if I worked out I could continue eating whatever I wanted, in whatever quantities I wanted. So, I continued eating junk, but working out hard in the gym, hoping I would lose weight. Guess what. After a year, I was even more overweight than I was before Not because of the exercise, but because I didn't watch what I was putting on my plate.

Here's a story that will show you that working out is not enough for weight loss. In the past, I was going for group exercise classes. Les Mills classes—really great, entertaining, fabulous classes. They are worldwide so you can check them out in your gym. Well, the group exercise instructors were usually doing class after class, having sometimes even 3 classes in the morning and 3 classes in the evening. They were burning tremendous amounts of energy each day, with a minimum of 700 hundred calories per class. Plus, if you add that to their BMR, the amount of energy they were burning per day was really very high. And yet, even though they were burning so many calories per day, some of them they were not completely trim. They had some extra fat. If you ask yourself how a person who is burning so much energy each day is not losing their extra fat, it's because they were not watching what is on their plate. It's that simple.

So, work out, but not more than an hour (unless you are a professional), and watch what you eat as well. Balance is the key.

Myth 3: You should work out on an empty stomach. There are many people out there that wake up in the morning and immediately go for a run or a workout on an empty stomach. There are just as many people out there who go as far as to promote this stuff. I completely disagree with it. This is not healthy at all because the body already is dehydrated and starved from so many hours of not eating or drinking during the night. (Read more about this in the chapter *Breakfast*.)

If you do this, you are going to put more pressure on your body by burning a lot of energy without any fuel, which is food. If you are thinking that in this way the body will burn fat, you are wrong, because the body will enter into starvation mode and instead store fat for use as energy later. Instead, it will burn energy from your muscles. And next time you eat, the body will store fat because your body believes you are going to keep it hungry and, on top of this, put high pressure on it with a workout on empty stomach.

My choice is this. Before I work out in the morning, I get a banana an hour before, or a slice of bread, and obviously water as soon as I wake up. But if you usually workout in the afternoon, then wait 2-3 hours after your lunch before you go for a workout, or even wait 4 hours before your workout if you had a very heavy lunch.

The idea is, don't start your workout hungry, but also don't start it with a full stomach.

Myth 4: Taking protein supplements will make you bulky. Not true. Taking proteins after your workout, if they are just basic proteins, will not make your muscles big and bulky. If you are doing weight training, I suggest after a workout to get some protein. This protein will help with the recovery of your muscles after a demanding workout.

My choice is, on the days that I lift weights, I take a low-fat protein shake after the workout. I usually buy the brands that have around 20 grams of protein, with a maximum of 200 calories per shake, but this is my choice. Research the subject, and make your choice. On the days I don't do weights and I do just cardio or a light yoga, I'll not take a protein shake, but usually I will eat a good meal after the workout.

So, the idea is, before a workout, eat some very light carbohydrates. This could be bread or a banana or dates or oats. There are many possibilities. The idea is to have some slow digesting carbohydrates. And after the workout, get some protein (a shake or a protein bar), or a healthy meal that has some protein in it, as well as healthy carbohydrates.

Don't forget, even if you work out, to stick to your weight loss daily calorie allowance.

What Might Keep You Overweight

1. Lack of sleep

There are two hormones that play an important role in your weight loss: leptin and ghrelin. These two hormones regulate your appetite and hunger.

Ghrelin is the hormone that tells you when to eat. When you are hungry you have more ghrelin than when you just finished eating.

Leptin is the hormone that tells you when you should stop eating.

When you are sleep deprived, that means you are not sleeping the minimum hours per day required for your age. The side effects of this are some hormonal disturbances of your ghrelin and leptin hormones. What exactly happens is, when you don't get enough sleep your body will have too much ghrelin and less leptin. You will be hungry more and you will be eating more. On top of that, the metabolism will be slower, because low leptin means that your body doesn't have enough energy stored, which will send a signal that you need to eat more and burn less.

So, if you have more ghrelin and less leptin you will for sure gain weight.

There is much research out there that clearly shows people who are sleep deprived gain weight.

So, I suggest get some proper sleep every night if you want to lose weight.

2. Soft drinks

Not only are they unhealthy, but they also have lots of sugar, with lots of calories. A big glass of soft drink can contain up to 250 calories, so why would you choose to drink your calories instead of eating them? Not to mention the health damage that this soft drink causes to your body.

If you want to drink some juice, choose fresh and choose the ones without sugar. You don't need extra sugar in your blood. It's not healthy, and it will lead to weight gain. Chose sugar-free juices, and also those not sweetened with any other chemicals. It might not taste as sweet, but it's much more healthy.

3. Alcohol

Not only does alcohol have calories, but also when it reaches your blood stream your metabolism slows down, and you will not lose any weight until the alcohol is out of your system. Because your body, instead of losing weight, is busy metabolizing the alcohol from your system.

4. Skipping meals

I talked in many chapters, even in the first one, about the importance of eating and not starving. If you don't eat your body is going to enter starvation mode, which will make you burn energy from your lean muscle and store fat next time you eat something. The same thing will happen if you skip meals.

Not only will your body enter starvation mode, but also ghrelin will increase, which will make you hungrier and make you eat more the next time you eat.

I wrote in a different chapter about my cousin who waited to eat when she was hungry. The more you wait the more ghrelin increases, but sometimes it's good to wait a little before you jump to eat at every hunger sensation. Just to be sure you are really hungry, not just angry or thirsty or any other feeling that might send you the signal that you are hungry. Learn to listen to your body and understand exactly what it wants.

Water and Vitamins

Water is essential. Why? First, your body needs it. But also, if you don't drink it, your brain sends you a thirst signal, which is very similar to the signal for hunger. However, your body cannot easily distinguish between thirst and hunger signals. Because of this, you might think you're hungry, when actually you're thirsty. And you will end up eating instead of drinking water, and this could cause overeating because you seem to be always hungry. Also, when you drink water, you burn more calories. Now please don't go crazy on the water. Just drink 2 to 3 liters (approximately 8 glasses) of water per day and no more.

Vitamins as well are essential for losing weight. When you're restricting your calorie intake, your body will not have enough food to get the amount of vitamins and minerals needed per day. Sometimes even if you eat normal amounts of food, the same thing can happen. So, you need to supplement your food with vitamins. Because if your body has a deficit of some vitamin, you might end up craving a certain food that your body knows it can get that vitamin from.

And forget about the myth that taking vitamins makes you fat or makes you hungry. It's just a myth. It's not true. So, get your supplement of vitamins and minerals now.

Centimeters (Inches) vs. Scale

So, you feel you lost some weight, and you go on a scale. What you see is a big disappointment. You didn't lose one gram (ounce), but somehow you feel yourself slimmer. How is it possible? Is your mind playing tricks? No, your mind is accurate. You did lose weight, but you lost in centimeters (inches). This is better, and here's why. Muscle is denser than fat. One kg (pound) of fat is much more in volume then one kg (pound) of muscle. To look slim in your clothes, it doesn't matter what you lose, fat or muscles. But to be healthy and look good naked you need to lose fat. Because it's the fat giving you that unaesthetic look, not the muscles. So, it's better to lose more in centimeters (inches) then in kg (pounds). If you want to measure your progress, weigh and measure yourself regularly, but not every day.

Take It Easy, Better Slow Than Never

We all want results now, maybe even yesterday, but fast results are not going to be sustainable. Because there are many implications, including psychological. If you have been overweight for many years, and in one month you become slim, it's going to be hard (but not impossible) for you to cope with. You suddenly have a new you that you don't know how to manage. You have a slim body, but an overweight identity. Everyone will tell you that you lost so much weight, but you will still consider yourself overweight. Yes, you will know that you lost weight, but in your mind, you will still be fat. Also, you didn't have the time to build a new lifestyle. If you lost weight so fast, probably it was not in a very healthy way. But if you give yourself time, to lose little by little, to get used to the new you every day, to build new habits, to be healthy, to accept the new you, then this will be sustainable. I've seen many people, myself included, when we lose weight fast we put it back fast. If you lose weight little by little every day, not only will your body change. You will change as well. And once you are slim, you will have had a terrific journey, during which you learned so much about yourself. And you will not go back to where you were.

My advice is: don't do anything that you will not do every day. For example, if you go to the gym because you want to lose weight and you stay there three hours, can you keep doing that every day? No, but maximum one hour per day you can do. So, build the habit for one hour and enjoy that one hour.

Another example, you eat only certain foods that are low in calories just so you can lose weight fast. Can you eat this way every day? No, you cannot. So, learn balance, every day, by eating what's right for the long term, not what makes you slim the fastest right now.

Don't be desperate for results. Just go slowly. Slow and sustainable. You will get results, and not just any results. You will get results that stay.

PART TWO

MIND

WEIGHT LOSS IS A MIND GAME

Strategies

Whether you are overweight right now or slim, it's because you have a strategy. Even if you don't realize it, this strategy is making you fat or keeping you slim.

I have a cousin who has always been slim. What I've noticed with many slim people is this. They don't necessarily have a better metabolism, although sometimes they do. Rather, most of the people that are slim are this way because they are simply eating less. To prove that, I started counting the calories my cousin ate. After counting for a few days, although her diet was full of chocolate and other delicious things, I noticed that rarely would she eat more than 1400 calories per day. One day she ate 2000 calories, but this is because it was her birthday celebration. Also, I noticed that she ate very slowly compared to me. On one of the occasions we spent together, we ate beans. She ate the beans with a fork, one by one, while I ate my beans with a spoon, 3 or 4 in one spoon. I finished in few minutes, but she took more than ten minutes to finish. One day she was very hungry and, although she was in the house and busily cooking food, she waited two hours before she sat down to eat something. Whereas when I was hungry, I would immediately pop some food in my mouth.

It is clearly a difference of strategy.

Now we can look back to the past and analyze why my cousin and I had different strategies, and I can point out where and how these differences came about. But that's not important. The idea is, if someone is successful at something, it means they have a good strategy.

We could say she has a good metabolism, but I doubt her metabolism is better than mine. Yet there is a difference, and it's this. She naturally eats less, which means fewer calories per day, but for me, I have to keep a close count so as not to eat more calories than I am allowed per day.

This was my cousin's strategy, although she was not aware she was using one. It's a strategy and a good one that could keep anyone fit.

So I thought, what if I took her strategy of keeping slim and implemented it on myself. For a week I started to eat like her. While eating beans, I ate one by one and slow. When I was hungry, I waited before I jumped to eat something. And I ate slowly. Now I was eating slowly by chewing the food more. In addition to this, I added also the strategy of Deepak Chopra of keeping fit, which is mindful eating. So, I was eating slower because I was chewing more, and while I was chewing I was really living in the moment without thinking about something else. Also, I didn't deny myself any type of food (which I never do anyway), but obviously the quantity was different.

What I noticed in a few days was like a miracle. My digestion was better, as I was eating slower and chewing food much more. Also, because I was being mindful of every piece of food I was eating, this made me eat way less. I started feeling overfull with half the quantity I was eating before.

And not only I was feeling fabulous with great energy, but my calorie intake was lower. Which was great.

Then one day I broke my new strategy and went back to eating more and faster. Over the next couple of days, I felt really sick. So, I decided to go back to my cousin strategy that was keeping her fit, trim, and slim, and I felt fabulous again. I still count calories as a habit, but I feel so much better.

The idea is, if you are overweight, ask yourself: what is your strategy? Because you do have one, even if you are not aware of it.

Then if you are fit, trim, slim, what's your strategy? If you have a good one, share it with others.

No matter what kind of body you have, just ask yourself what strategy are you using to have the body that you have right now. And if you would like to improve your body, ask yourself, what strategy do I need to adopt that will make my body fit, trim, slim?

You can for sure apply the strategy outlined in this book, but if you think that something else will work for you, go for that instead. Do what you feel is right for you. Listen to yourself and to your body.

The strategy presented in this book, I find to be the easiest and healthiest, as it is not suppressing you from anything.

Likewise, you can ask people who have the body that you want what their strategy is. What do they do in order to achieve this result? And use them as a model. Also, find out what they believe about themselves, about weight loss, about having a fit, trim body. And if their beliefs resonate with you, embrace them and make them your own beliefs. Make them your programs. (Our mental programs are discussed in the chapter *Affirmations*.)

Find the strategy you are currently using. Modify it. If it makes sense, apply the strategy outlined in this book, or find another strategy that works for you. And become a person with the body you always wanted to have. A slim, fit, trim body.

The Power of Focus and Goals

We keep hearing: goals, goals, goals! Make goals! It's kind of annoying, isn't it? But it is helpful, and here's why.

Whatever you tell your brain is what it's going to focus on. For example, if I tell you today to go outside and notice how many red cars there are, you will suddenly start seeing more red cars. Then if I tell you to go and see how many yellow cars there are, you will suddenly see yellow cars everywhere. And you will see more than red. Because this is what you told your brain to do.

Now, goals are simple and effective ways of telling your brain what you want to see and get. The brain, in response, is working for you to accomplish that. For example, let's say you tell your brain, I want to lose weight. This is how much I want to lose, and you keep saying this every day. Then, in reply to your new goal, the brain is going to focus to help you lose weight. Suddenly you will not have the same appetite. Suddenly you will find more ways to reach your goal faster. A lot of things will change that will support you in achieving your goal. But your brain needs to know what you want. So, tell it what you want. Tell it exactly the number you want to lose, and remind it every day and night what your goal is. It will help you accomplish it in the fastest and easiest way. Just trust it. The brain's capacity is unlimited. You just need to put it to good use.

Raise Your Standards

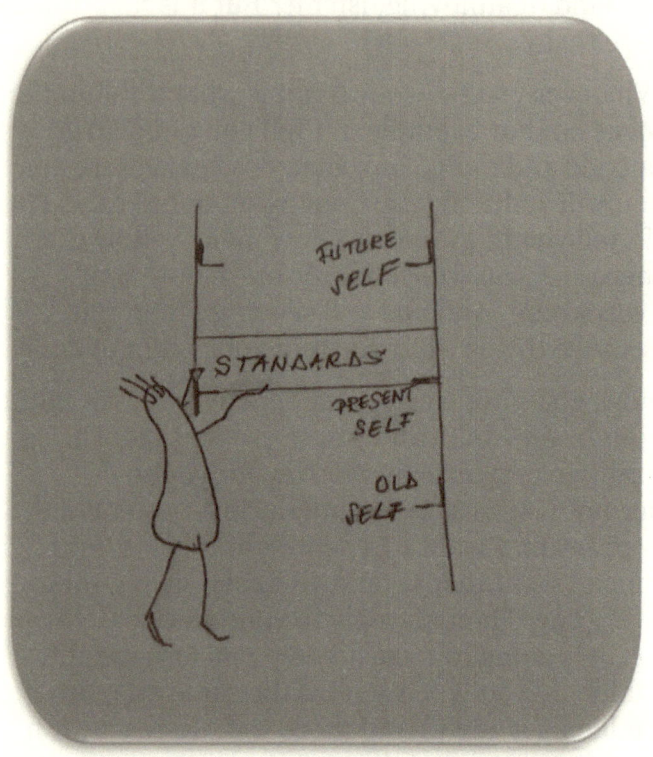

There are people out there who are always in fabulous shape no matter what is happening in their life. Problems, stress, work issues, kid issues, pregnancies, diseases, etc. They don't miss workouts, they eat clean.

What's the difference between these people who look great and put in great effort no matter what, and others who don't?

The difference is in their standards. They have high standards for their health and their body. They have high expectations for themselves. They demand from themselves and from their bodies much more than you demand if you are not in the same great shape.

I remember I had a friend in school, and she was always very careful about what she was eating, when I was not. From any standard, she was slim and I was overweight. Still, she would be preoccupied with what she was putting in her mouth, and I wouldn't be. I went to her home one day, and there in the bedroom she had a stationary bicycle, which she would ride almost every day. She even had in her home a lot of sweets, which she was kind enough to offer me. She ate also, but not as much as I did. She took just a piece. Although she wanted more, she didn't take more. I did. A few years down the line, I was fatter and she was fitter. It took me a few years to understand what the difference is between her and me. We both craved, we both didn't like to do sports, but one of us, even though she was still craving, was able to control herself, and would do sports even if it was not enjoyable.

What was the difference between her and me? Why was she so healthy and conscientious, and I was not?

The difference was in our standards. One of us, me at that time, had low standards for my body and health, while my friend had very high standards.

This is the difference between those who look great and those who don't. Many can do it, but only few choose to do it.

So in order to have a trim, fit, slim body, you must raise your standards, and you must change what you accept from yourself and what you don't accept from yourself anymore. Don't tolerate overeating any longer. Don't tolerate junk food anymore. Demand more from yourself and from your body. What you tolerate you become, so don't tolerate anything that is unhealthy, that doesn't nourish you, that doesn't empower you, that doesn't help your health and wellbeing.

Set your standards high, from what you eat to what activities you do.

Fit, trim, slim should be the standard of your body for life. If you don't make this your standard, fit, trim and slim will never be sustainable.

Visualization

Law of Reversed Effort: "When the will and the imagination are in conflict, the imagination invariably wins the day." (Émile Coué)

Now that you have your goal written on a paper, I want you to imagine how you would look at that certain weight. How you would feel. What you would hear. Imagine yourself reaching your goal, being that fit, slim, trim person you've wanted to be for so long. Imagine it, feel it, hear it, see it, live it. And do this every morning and evening. Even during the day, the more you visualize the better. The more you visualize, the more you remind your brain about your goal, the faster you will achieve it.

Visualization is one of the most important things you can do for everything you desire. If you can see it in your mind, you can create it with your body, but if you cannot see it, it is very difficult for you to create it. And I'm talking about any outcome. Most people who did great things in life saw first what they wanted to achieve in their mind. However, to really let your mind flow and be able to truly see things that are not there (but things that you want to happen), you need to reach a meditative state. In this state, your conscious mind is sleeping and you have full access to the most powerful mind that is responsible for almost everything happening in your body and behavior. This is your subconscious mind.

If you don't know how to enter in this meditative

state, this is how you do it. Note that this is just one example. There are so many ways of doing it. Feel free to adjust it according to your preferences.

Find a comfortable position. I personally prefer lying down, but you can choose sitting in the lotus position or on a chair or sofa. The bottom line is that you need to sit comfortable and relax. Make sure you are alone in the room and that for the next 10-15 minutes no one will disturb you. Make sure you have your phone on silent mode.

Sit, close your eyes and relax, take few deep, slow breaths. After you finish with this, start counting from 50 backwards. While you are counting try to visualize the number that you are counting. 50 and visualize 50, 49 and visualize 49 . . . and so on until you reach 0. There are other ways to enter this meditative state, but if you are a beginner, this is the easiest. Please make sure to count slowly. If you are lying down, it's possible for you to feel so deeply relaxed that you might fall asleep. If this happens, next time choose one of the comfortable sitting positions.

When you have finished counting, you will be very relaxed. Now start using your creativity and picture yourself slim. If you cannot picture yourself slim, just ask yourself, how would I look if I were to be slim, fit, trim, and wait for the answer while trying again to see yourself in that great shape. In a few seconds the picture will come into your mind, and you will start admiring yourself. See what clothes you will wear, how happy you will be, and just go ahead create great memories with you in that great shape. Let your imagination flow. Do this for a few minutes, and then after you really see yourself in that great shape and you've created some wonderful memories, go into your body, into your new fit, trim, slim body, and live in that moment. Imagine what you will see, what you will hear, what you will feel. If it's difficult for you to picture yourself in your great body, ask yourself, how would I feel, what would I hear and what would I see if I were already fit, trim, slim. Then let your imagination flow again. Feel really great. Feel like it's all real. Let go of everything and just live the moment like it's real, like it's happening right now.

Do this visualization for as long as you want, and when you want to come out of this state, tell yourself, I'm going to count from 0 to 5, and at 5 I'm going to open my eyes, and I'm going to feel great, full of energy and vitality, and I'm going to have a great day. And open your eyes.

Do this as many times as you can, but you must do it at least once a day.

Affirmations

What you tell yourself over and over is what your mind is going to believe is the truth. The mind doesn't understand jokes. For example, if you tell yourself over and over that it's very hard to lose weight, guess what, your subconscious mind is going to believe it and is going to make this a fact, which will make your weight loss very hard. This weight loss difficulty can come by having a lot of urges to eat more than you should, by struggling to keep to your daily calorie goal, and in many other ways. That will make this weight loss journey very hard because your belief is that it is very hard to lose weight.

But if you tell yourself that it's effortless to lose weight, then you will find the strategies mentioned here very easy to apply, and you will lose weight easy and fast. This is because you have the belief that it's effortless to lose weight.

To explain why, understand that our main behavior comes not from our conscious mind, but rather from our subconscious mind. The subconscious mind is the part of your mind that manages all bodily functions, like keeping your heart beating, and all your other organs functioning properly. You don't tell yourself to start your heart beating. The subconscious mind does it for you. But this subconscious mind is running on programs. For example, if you tell yourself you would like to lose weight, you are saying it at the conscious level. But at the same time, you find yourself eating more, and you

---

cannot control this eating. This is because at a subconscious level you have a program that is overpowering your desire at a conscious level to lose weight. It's kind of a battle. You want to lose weight in your conscious mind, but if your subconscious mind is not aligned with this desire then you are not going to lose weight. Because most of your behavior is driven by your subconscious mind. You don't tell your heart to beat. And even if you tried to do this with your conscious mind, your subconscious mind would still do what it knows best and what it's programed to do.

So, in order to align your conscious mind (which is your desire to lose weight) with the subconscious mind (your behavior), you need to align both parts of your mind on the same page. In order to do that, you need to program your subconscious mind for weight loss success.

If you are overweight right now, most likely you have programed your subconscious mind to keep you overweight. If you tell your conscious mind that you've decided to lose weight, but your subconscious mind is programmed to keeping you overweight, you will see in your behavior that it will be very difficult for you to lose weight. You will have constant cravings. You will not be able to control your calories. And if you lose a little weight, you will sabotage yourself with days of feasting.

If order for you to have success in your weight loss journey, you need to program your conscious mind, but even more so your subconscious mind, for success.

To do that, you need to install new programs. As I said earlier, what you tell your mind through repetition, your mind will believe to be true, and this will show itself in your behavior.

So, if you've continuously told yourself over the years that you can't lose weight, or that it's hard to lose weight (because that has been your experience so far), then that is exactly what you will encounter now, no matter how easy the new strategy is. In the same way, if you've continuously told yourself that you're fat, then you have believed it to be true, and it's going to keep you fat. (Read more about this in the chapter *Your Identity*.)

So, to succeed in any weight loss journey, you have to make your mind believe things that it doesn't currently believe, like telling to yourself that weight loss is easy and effortless for you. I'm sure when you read this, you said in your mind: No, it's not true. But through repetition, even if it's not true, you will start to believe it, and you will start acting like it. For example, start telling to yourself right now: Weight loss comes effortlessly to me; I lose weight fast and easy. And read this over a few times. At the beginning, you read it, and your conscious mind said: No, it's not true. But if you continuously say this affirmation, you will slowly start believing it, and slowly start acting like it. Then gradually it will become a truth for you. Once it becomes a truth for you, that means it has entered your subconscious mind as a program, and you will start noticing the results. Losing weight will become really easy and effortless because this is the new program your subconscious mind is running, and this is what is going to show up in your body. As I said, you don't tell your heart to beat. The subconscious mind does it for you. Likewise, the subconscious mind will make you slim.

Now in order to have programs that lead you to a successful weight loss story, and in order to sustain it, you need to install even more programs in your subconscious mind. These programs are affirmations that are going to lead you to success. You can add more, but here are some:

The past does not equal the future. I took this from Tony Robbins's book, and I find it a very powerful program for your weight loss journey, and for your life. Because our brain tends to generalize everything in order to give us a sense of certainty, and it tends to think that if in the past I didn't succeed then I'm less likely to succeed in the future, which is not a good program to run. So, in order for the brain not to create this generalization (which we all do), this affirmation will help you a lot. If you were not successful in the past on your weight loss journey, it doesn't mean that now you will not be successful. So, repeat over and over ... *The past does not equal the future* ... until it becomes a truth for you.

Other affirmations: *I can do and achieve whatever my mind can conceive.*

One of my favorites, also from Tony Robbins's book, *Nothing tastes as good as thin feels.*

Having this affirmation, as a belief will make your mind prioritize keeping you fit over eating any delicious food you might encounter. Like, if you have a chocolate and you want to eat it all when you see it, but you have this belief that *Nothing tastes as good as thin feels*, your mind will stop you from eating all the chocolate. You will have the power to eat only a few pieces, and the rest you will share it, or keep it for another day, because your mind will prioritize feeling thin much more than the feeling of chocolate on your taste buds. And you will make this choice effortlessly. It will come naturally for you, even if your whole life you ate all the chocolate and you couldn't control yourself. Now you will be able to control your cravings, and it will be such a natural thing, as though you've been doing it forever.

Being fit, trim, slim is safe. Changing the way we look may sometimes make us feel unsafe at an unconscious level. And if we feel unsafe at an unconscious level, we might tend to start eating, to have cravings, and we won't know why. This might be the reason. So tell yourself ... *it's safe to be fit, trim, slim* ... over and over.

Losing weight is easy and effortless.

I am slim, fit and trim. Even though you don't believe it and you're not there yet, it's a must for you to say this. Because when your subconscious mind will believe it, it will give you the behavior of a slim, fit, trim person. (Read more about this in the chapter *Your Identity*.)

Eating healthy food in the right quantity makes

me feel great.

Exercising makes me feel great and alive. Once you believe this, going for a workout is not going to be a dread anymore. It will be something you look forward to.

Fit, trim, and slim is the way to be for life.

I am safe, all is well. This is one of the most important affirmations because sometimes when we are going through stressful periods we tend to eat more, have crazy cravings, and have difficulty continuing with any weight loss program. To avoid this, if you feel down, or stressed, or you notice that you want to eat more and more, just repeat this affirmation, over and over every day, until the stressful period is gone. You will see that saying this affirmation will affect you immediately, and it will release you from crazy cravings. This affirmation is one of the few, which you might need to say for your whole life, whenever stressful situations appear, or while facing difficulties in your life. It is very useful, not only for weight loss but for your internal peace as well. Remember ... *I am safe, all is well.*

These are some of the affirmations that I suggest you use in your weight loss journey. Don't just say them. You must believe them, even if you don't believe them now. They are going to take you where you want to be: a fit, trim, slim person for life. Just do it.

For things to change, you must change. And what you must change are the programs you are currently running that are stopping you from losing weight.

Make your brain and your mind work for you.

Rewards

I've noticed something about a lot of people when they are on a diet. After they lose few kg (pounds), to celebrate this small success, or big success, they celebrate it with food. A lot of food, which usually on their weight loss journey they would not eat, or which they would eat only in small quantities. But now, in celebrating their success, they go out and eat anything and everything.

Know that this kind of celebration is going to take you backward, to regain the weight you lost.

Going out to celebrate your new healthy behavior, that is leading you to success, with an old unhealthy behavior that led you to having a weight problem, is definitely going to affect your weight loss success in the future. You should not reinforce good, healthy behavior with unhealthy, destructive behavior.

If you want to celebrate your weight loss success, which I absolutely encourage you to do, try this instead. Set small goals and big goals before you start, and throughout your weight loss journey. Every time you reach these milestones, decide in advance that you will reward yourself with maybe new clothes, or a day at the spa, or something really nice that will make you feel good about yourself and about your success. Reaching these goals, and rewarding yourself for them, will make you want to lose weight more, and you will have more and more success. But remember that rewards should never be food. Under no circumstances should you reward your weight loss with food.

Because if you do, you will be teaching yourself the wrong thing.

In your weight loss journey you are not only going to lose weight. While you are doing it, you are also changing the behavioral patterns that made you gain weight. When these behavioral patterns change, you will never have a weight problem again. That's why it is very important not to reward yourself with food. Because if you do this, these unhealthy behaviors will never change. And if they never change, you will never be able to sustain your weight loss, and you will go back to the person you no longer want to be, an overweight person.

Remember you are not on a diet. You are on a journey to change your lifestyle, which is going to reward you by building the fit, trim, body that you want.

So, reward yourself with anything but food, and you will create a lifestyle that will keep you fit, trim, slim for life.

Your Identity

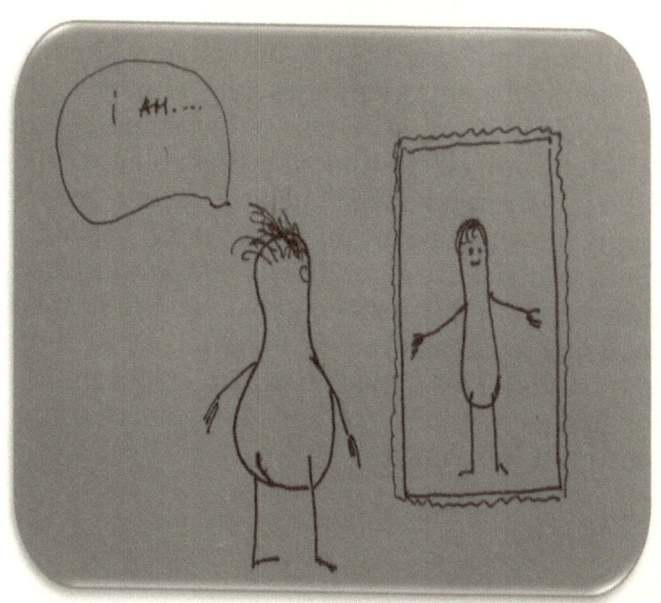

When you were overweight, your mind knew you were overweight. You built your identity around it. If I were to ask you to give a description of yourself that included your body, you would tell me you were overweight.

But after a diet, if I were to ask you if you're slim, somehow, you would still tell me you need to lose weight. Why does this happen, and what will happen if you don't change it?

This happens because you've lived so many years being overweight, so your mind, no matter how slim you are, still sees you like this.

But you must change it. And this is because, if you are slim but have an identity of being overweight, you will become overweight again. It's just a matter of time, but it will happen.

From now on, I want you to build a new identity for yourself, a new identity as a fit, slim, trim person. And it's so easy. One of the things you can do is tell yourself continuously that you are slim. Even if your mind doesn't believe it, continue saying it over and over until your mind has no doubt that you are slim. Even if you want to lose more kg (pounds), believing that you are slim is not going to change your motivation to lose more kg (pounds). Lie to your mind. Trick your mind, and make it happen. You are slim, you are trim, you are fit, yes you are!

Six Basic Human Needs

There are six basic human needs. We all have them, and the way we prioritize them determines how we behave. The six basic human needs are:

The need for certainty: to know for sure that you have what you need for basic survival, like food and shelter, to know for sure that you are financially safe, to know for sure that you are loved unconditionally, etc.

The need for variety: Tony Robbins in his seminars, when he is explaining this need, asks a question: Do you love surprises? And the whole room usually says, yes! And then he replies: Bullshit! You love the surprises you want. The other ones you call problems!

Also, he mentions that God gave you this second need for variety because he knew that if you had only certainty you would be bored out of your senses. And this is true. If you knew at every moment what was going to happen, and you were certain about that, life would not be fun or entertaining. You would be so bored. So, God, as Tony Robbins says, gave this second need for variety, which is also uncertainty: the need for surprises, for change, for new things and new experiences. That's why most of us love to travel, because it gives us tremendous variety.

The third need is *the need for connection and love:* as the Dalai Lama said, "we are all social beings," and we will not be happy without each other.

But we need more from each other. We need to feel connected and feel loved and give love.

The forth need is *the need for significance:* we all need to feel important at some level, we all need to feel unique and special.

The fifth and the sixth needs are the needs of the spirit. These are the most fulfilling ones and these are: *the need of contribution and growth*.

We all have the need to contribute to others beyond our means. This fulfills us in a beautiful way. When you give to a person a gift, and that gift is received so wonderfully, you feel much better than the person who received it. Or, if you ever helped someone with a big problem, solving his or her problem not only made the other person happy, it also made you feel so fulfilled.

As for the last one, *the need for growth:* there is this law of nature—if something is not growing it's dying. And this is one of the most fulfilling needs in life because growth is progress, and when you make progress in any area of your life, it's a tremendously fulfilling experience.

Now as I said at the beginning, the way we prioritize them determines how we act. Note that we are fulfilling all these needs at any given moment, even if we are not aware of it, and we fulfill them in either a positive or a negative way. Each one of us, prioritize two of this needs more than the others.

Let me give you an example: I give the highest priority to growth. This is number one for me.

Now everything I do at any given moment, I do to fulfill all my needs, but growth in particular. That's why one of my biggest hobbies is reading. This not only fulfills my need for growth but is also fulfilling my need for significance. It makes me feel that I belong to a group of intellectual people, and it meets my need for connection because I can connect with people and talk about the latest things I've read. This fulfills my need for variety because I don't know exactly what I am going to learn while reading the book, and it fulfills my need for certainty that I'm going to learn something for sure. In turn, this fulfills my need for contribution because what I learn I can immediately apply on my clients, friends, family to help them better their lives. This is just an example of how an activity fulfills my first basic human need, as well as how it fulfills my other basic human needs.

Now if there is something that you enjoy doing it is because it fulfills most of your basic human needs at a very high level.

If I would to ask you about your hobby, or an activity that you enjoy doing, on a scale of 0 to 10, 0 being the minimum and 10 being the maximum, how much does this activity fulfill your need for certainty, variety, connection and love, significance, contribution and growth?

I bet it's fulfilling all yours needs at a very high scale.

Now look at something that you don't enjoy doing, and I am sure that activity will not be fulfilling your basic human needs at a very high level.

Let me give you my example for an activity that I don't enjoy doing. For me, it's cooking. Although I believe I'm a good cook, I enjoy cooking only occasionally. Let see how cooking fulfills my basic human needs. How much growth do I have when I cook: maybe a 5 if I invent some new dish, but if it's a food that I've cooked before then it's a 2. How does cooking fulfill my certainty? Maybe an 8, because I'm certain I know how to cook and I'm going to have edible results. It might be good. I know I might not enjoy doing the dishes after however, so an 8. How about my need for variety? I'd say 4, because there's not variety in it. Even if I cook different food, I don't get much variety from it. How about my need for significance? Probably 3. I am just a normal cook so it doesn't give me much significance either. Connection? Maybe a 6, if I cook for someone who enjoys my cooking. But this would not be every day. And contribution? Maybe a 7, if I also cook for someone. Otherwise, both of them are under 5.

So, having these levels of fulfillment of my basic human needs, no wonder I don't enjoy cooking, but I very much enjoy reading. Because reading fulfills my needs at a very high level. There are people out there for whom cooking fulfills them highly. I heard even of people for whom cleaning fulfills them at a very high level, but I'm not one of them.

This happens with everything in your life, be it with people, activities, and your job. The more needs are fulfilled by an activity or a person, the more pleasurable it will be, and the more you will enjoy it. And the opposite is true when there is less need for an activity or person. That fulfills you at a very low level, and is less pleasurable.

What does this have to do with food? Well, a lot. Because food fulfills all your basic human needs at a very high level, and if something is fulfilling more than 3 basic human needs, it becomes an addiction. And food is an addiction anyway, but it's an addiction that we need for survival.

The same happens with drugs and alcohol and smoking. These fulfill more than 3 of your needs at a very high level, so they become an addiction.

Let's go back to food and see how it fulfills each of your basic human needs.

Food and certainty: Food fulfills your need of certainty at a very high level because you know it's available, you know it's going to make you feel good, you know it's tasty, and you know that you can eat it.

Food and variety: I'm sure you are not eating the same thing at every meal, so you have many options to choose from: from sweet to sour to salty, different cuisines, different dishes, which you can eat from different restaurants, places etc.; Food therefore provides you with a tremendous variety at a very high level.

Food and connection: Sharing food with someone and eating together gives you a tremendous sense of connection, that's why there are dinner dates!

Food and significance: If you eat healthy, you get a sense of belonging and significance that you belong to a group of people who watch what they eat and are healthy and fit. On the other hand, if you eat unhealthy and you are sick, you'll have a sense of belonging to that category of people who have weight and health problems. Both ways will give you a high level of significance, belonging and connection at the same time.

Food and growth: You can grow by having a healthy lifestyle and being more energetic and alive through the healthy food you eat, or you can grow in size if you eat unhealthily. You are growing both ways so your need of growth is fulfilled at a very high level.

Food and contribution: You can give other people some of your food or buy food for someone else and this will give you a high level of contribution.

Now you have seen how food can fulfill your basic human needs at a very high level. But the way we use food is different. As you can see above, some people use food in a positive empowering way and some people use food in a destructive way.

Note: We make the decisions to fulfill our needs at a subconscious level but now that we know about them, we can make them conscious by bringing them to our awareness.

Now, I'm going to talk about those people who are using food in a destructive way, like overeating, or eating only junk.

The people who eat junk or overeat don't do it

every day (a very few of them do it daily because they don't know better), but most of them only do it sometimes. Maybe they eat unhealthy every day but they don't always self-load to destruction. The moments that they do overeat or self-load with food are the moments when their basic human needs are not fulfilled, so they found this negative way to fulfill them.

As I said before, the decision to fulfill the needs, which are not met and meet them in a different way through an empowering or destructive way are done at a subconscious level.

How many people have you heard who are overeating while stressed? This is because if they are stressed, probably some of their basic human needs are not being fulfilled at a very high level so they turn to food to fulfill their needs.
It's a tradition in the movies, when a girl breaks up with a boy, she starts eating ice cream. What would happen if this were real? In some cases, it is real. What happens, the girl that suffers from the breakup does not feel certain about her future love life. She does not feel connected or loved. She might be feeling insignificant so she turns to ice cream because the ice cream will fulfill some of her needs that must be fulfilled in that moment.
I have personally seen many ladies who were slim before their marriage and after their marriage, they started to pack on a huge amount of weight. What happened? Did they just suddenly decide to eat more? No. They are just unhappy and unfulfilled and if their needs are not fulfilled in the relationship with their husband, then they

usually turn to food to fulfill those unmet needs. Food is a very easy and accessible way to fulfill your unmet needs.

Let me tell you, no person gains weight without a reason, and no person keeps the weight without a reason. When I work with a new client, I ask: When did you start gaining weight? What happened in that period? Because I know something happened. People don't just gain weight without a reason and most of the time, the reason is psychological. And if that psychological reason is not solved, weight loss might be difficult.

For example, no matter if you are a women or a men, and you gained a big amount of weight, what I would suggest is to find out what made you gain weight in the first place and what is the real reason that you turned to food. In which circumstances do you turn to food for comfort? When do you engage in bingeing? What is your mental state in that exact moment that makes you turn to food? And as a solution, I suggest in that moment, when you are just about to fulfill your unmet needs with food to find another way than food to fulfill these needs. As well ask yourself, am I hungry for food or am I hungry for something else?
Moreover, if something is not fulfilling your needs in the long term, you need to make a change. If your needs are not being met and you always choose to take the easiest way to fulfill your needs with food or cigarettes or alcohol, then you need to look at the main problem that is causing all

this, and try to solve it. Look also for alternative ways to fulfill your needs in an empowering way. Yes, food will always fulfill your needs, but use it for survival and use it to fulfill your needs in an empowering way, like getting significance from belonging to the healthy category of people. Take variety from the variety of healthy food. Take certainty from food by eating the right food that is going to build the body you desire. Take connection by connecting with people who share the same healthy goals as yours. Fulfill your growth need by having a better and healthier body every day and so on. Don't use food to make yourself feel good. When you can't feel good, find something else that can fulfill your needs and make you feel good in that moment.

I suggest making a list with all the things that make you feel good, and I'm sure there are plenty, such as going for a movie, riding your car, going to the gym, or listening to music, and make this list as long as possible, and when you feel down, instead of going for food, go to the list and do one of the activities that makes you feel good, and you will see that your overeating will disappear. Another suggestion is, don't eat if you are angry, feeling down or feeling hopeless, don't eat until you start feeling better. Do something to shift your mind, and when you feel better then eat, because if you eat when you are down or sad, you will be eating to make yourself better which you should not do, because if you are sad or down, that's because your needs are not fulfilled. Fulfill your needs in ways other than food, and then when you feel better, you can go and eat if you are hungry.

Conclusion: at any given moment, you are fulfilling your basic human needs. If it's something you enjoy, it fulfills your needs at a high level, if it's something that you don't enjoy, it fulfills your needs at a low level.
But there are some things that you can do to increase the level of how an activity fulfills you. Let's take an example like running, if you don't enjoy running like me, ask yourself: What do I need to do in order to increase the level of certainty while running? Then you do the same for variety, then significance, then connection, then growth and contribution, and write down at least three answers to each basic need and apply them. I'm sure that if you do this, the activity you didn't enjoy that much, like me with running can become an activity that you will start enjoying. But do this only if you want to.

But there is something that you need to do. You need to do the same example from above, but do it with eating healthy, working out and having a healthy lifestyle. If all these three are fulfilling you already at a very high level then there's no need to do it, however if are not, then do it, because in order for things to change, you need to find new ways to change.

Love Your Neighbour as Yourself

"Love your neighbor as you love yourself."
(Matthew 22:39)

What does this have to do with weight loss? A lot. Read through to the end, and you'll see why.

The problem with *Love your neighbor as you love yourself* is this. We might love our neighbor, and we might even love our neighbor *more* then we love our self. Because most of us go our whole life *without* love for our self.

This is because we have perfection standards, and unless we achieve them, we are incapable of love and compassion for ourselves. These perfection standards most likely start with the body that we have. We must have a certain body. We must look a certain way before we even start to consider ourselves worthy of love.

I'm here to tell you that having these perfection standards show that you really have no standard because *perfection doesn't exist*. There is no person in this world that can attain all these standards. But, in the eyes of the creator, we are all perfect.

No matter which size you are, no matter how you look, if you don't love yourself now as you are, you are not going to love yourself later. Even if you lose all the weight you want to lose.

I have someone close to me who unfortunately was in an accident that left him with many scars.

79

This is very unfortunate for someone to go through this incredible emotional and physical pain. What is more painful is having to watch this wonderful man, who has gone through so much pain, now going through the additional pain of not accepting what has happened and striving for perfection through multiple plastic surgeries.

The solution to this is not to seek perfection through plastic surgery. Because even if he will get the perfection he's striving for, it will not be truly fulfilling in the end. He will have the perfect body, but still will not be at peace with himself or love himself. Because love is not found on the outside though achievement. It's found on the inside. In fact, we are born with it.

When we were babies, we loved everything about ourselves. We even loved our poop. We fascinated ourselves, but then society told us, while we were growing up, that we were not good enough. We needed to be certain way to be worthy of love, even from ourselves. From that moment, we spent our lives searching for ways to achieve perfection so we could reach back to the state of love we once felt.

Because it's all about love. Life is all about love. We want to achieve because we think more people will love us more. We want to look a certain way because we think we will get more love, and so on.

If you want to look a certain way, if it's not for health or wellbeing, if it's just for vanity, then you are doing it because at the subconscious level you believe that only then will you be good enough.

And if you are good enough, you are worthy of love.

But what if you decide that you are good enough right now, and love yourself as you are right now? How do you think you would feel, and how will this impact your interaction with others? I'm telling you, it's going to feel so fulfilling, and you will finally be at peace. You will know that, no matter what, you are worthy of love.

Even if you have 100 kg (220 pounds) to lose, you should still start with loving yourself as you are right now, and start losing weight because you care and love yourself so much that you believe your health is important. Once you do that, you will feel fulfilled from day one. And once you are at a healthy weight, you will feel fabulous. Because you will be healthy, not because you will be living up to the standards of society.

Once you find the love for yourself on the inside, you will radiate it through to the outside.

There is no such thing as perfection. Even the ladies from the magazines don't really look the way they are portrayed there. They're wearing lots of makeup, and their pictures are airbrushed with Photoshop. Those are unrealistic standards. I was in a magazine, and my photo was airbrushed also. I know because all the moles (beauty spots, I like to call them) where not in the photo, but in reality I have them. Did I choose to airbrush my photo? No. The magazine did. It's their standard. They have to do it in order to sell because other magazines they do it also. So, everyone must do it.

Because in the society that we live in today, people tell you that who you are is not good enough. So you have to pretend to be someone you are not, and you have to start working toward becoming someone who is perfect. And that's something you will never achieve because perfection doesn't exist.

If you're reading this book to lose weight because of health reasons, then use it. But if you want to lose weight because you are hoping you will finally accept yourself once you live up to the unrealistic standards of society that you see in magazines, this book will not make that happen. It will be helpful to lose weight, but it will not be helpful in making you happy or in helping you to accept yourself and love yourself. Because no matter how good you look, by itself that will never be enough.

So, start with thinking that you are enough. Start loving yourself as you are, the wonderful being that you are. Who cares if you have some cellulite! Jillian Michael, although she is so toned and trim, admitted she has cellulite on her butt. So what if you don't have a body like the ones in magazines! You have a body, it's yours, and it deserves your love and acceptance.

No matter how many kg (pounds) you have to lose, please embark on this weight loss journey for the right reasons. Do it for health, for energy, for yourself, but not for unrealistic standards.

You Can Do It, The Past Does Not Equal the Future

Have you ever heard stories of people who were total nobodies for half their life, people no one ever believed would do big things in their lives, but then out of the blue they started doing truly remarkable things and are now changing people's lives for the better? Have you ever heard of people like this?

Or, have you ever heard of someone who was totally unhealthy, obese, with no will power or determination, living a totally sedentary life, and no one believed they would ever get better, but suddenly that person made a decision to change their life, and turned their whole life around, lost weight, became healthy and, along with this, became an example for society that it's possible and that there is still hope? If you by any chance haven't heard of these examples you don't need to look far, because a high number of people who write books, promote nutrition and a healthy lifestyle, are people who one day were helpless and no one believed they could succeed in losing weight, not to mention becoming so successful that they can, by themselves, inspire and help other people change their lives. Some of the biggest self-help gurus are people who at one time couldn't help themselves. I was one of them. I know many people whose life transformation astonished me, and I thought if they could do it so can I. If it's possible in the world, then it's possible for me, and it is possible for you also. It's only a matter of how.

If you are reading this book and you are in an unhealthy state where you are overweight and have lots of health problems, where you are using food in a destructive way, where you've tried so many things but you couldn't do it, know there is still hope for you. And there is still hope for you in a big way, because the things you are struggling with today might be the same things that make you successful tomorrow, if only you find a way to solve them. This experience will help you connect with, and understand, people who are going through same things, and you will be able to help them because you know how, you did it yourself. And if you can do it, others can as well. At that point, not only will you have changed your life, but also your changing will have a positive impact on the lives of so many other people. I don't know who you might be tomorrow. You might still be overweight and unhealthy, but there is a very high change you will be healthy and successful. Anything is possible.

What I want you to understand from this is that it doesn't matter who you were in the past, what you did or what you are currently doing right now. These things don't determine who you will be in the future. But what you are going to do tomorrow determines who you will be in the future, and even tomorrow might not count so much because soon it will be yesterday. The idea is, don't lose hope, and keep doing what is right. You will reach your goal, sooner or later, but if you bought this book it will be sooner because that shows that you have the desire to make it happen. And once you have this desire, you will find the ways and the tools to reach there.

I would be more than happy to hear about you one day, to hear that you have become a health guru, or a self-help guru, who once had a hard life and an unhealthy body but who changed it and now is an inspiration. Allow me to hear from you. Give yourself this wonderful gift that is going to be passed on to generations to come. Whoever you are out there reading this, no matter where you come from or what your circumstances, I BELIEVE IN YOU. Even though I don't know you and even though no one ever believed in you. Because if you were put on this earth by the creator (whoever you think that is), the creator would not put you here without all the tools you need to succeed, which are not different than mine, yours or any other being. You can do it.

You can do it. For sure you can. The past does not equal the future.

PART THREE

AFTER

100-Day Challenge

To recap, here's what you need to do.

As soon as you decide what your goal weight is, do the following:

1. Love yourself!

2. Calculate your BMR.

3. Get a list of the calories in foods and activities. Or, if you have a smartphone, there are some very nice apps, which can calculate all day long how many calories you eat and burn. The app I used to enjoy using was *Myfitnesspal*, as it has most of the foods and products with calories listed there. Also, I'm sure there are many other good apps on the market right now, so pick which one you think is most suitable for you.

4. Decide how many calories you will eat and what activities you will do, and make a plan for a healthy weight loss journey.

5. Raise your standards.

6. Visualize daily, and read your goals.

7. Use daily affirmations.

8. Change your identity.

9. Get vitamins.

10. Drink plenty of water.

11. Reward yourself.

12. Most importantly, believe you can do it, because if you can believe it, you can achieve it.

After you lose weight:

1. Decide your daily calorie intake.

2. Make a sustainable plan for a healthy balanced life.

Many years back, I was watching a show, I think on MTV, where people who were overweight were taking the *100-day challenge*.

They were given a personal trainer and they were taught what they had to do to lose weight, but it was up to them to follow it. The challenge would start from *Day 100* till *Day 0*. They would have a big calendar on the wall where *Day 100* was written as the start day and every day, they would rip up the page from the previous day, until they reached *Day 0*. On *Day 0*, they were supposed to reach their goal, whatever that healthy goal would be in that amount of time.

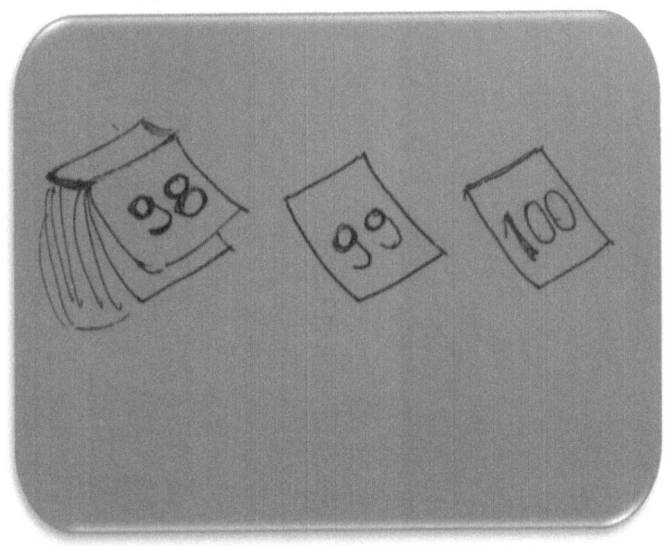

Now, I challenge you to give yourself *100 days* to reach a reasonable goal. Don't put "lose 30 kg in 100 days", because it's not healthy to lose that fast. Give yourself these *100 days*, where you will workout 5 times a week, you will eat healthy 80% of your food, you will stay in your daily calories allowance, and you will learn and use new strategies that would help you lose weight and sustain it. You will do affirmations, and you will follow what is outlined in this book. You could add more things that you would like to do in these *100 days*. The goal is to build new habits and lose weight. You should also put the exact number of kg or pounds you would like to lose in these *100 days*, a weight that is healthy for you to lose.

I am planning to make a group for all the people who read this book and are interested in having some support in this *100-day challenge*. If you are one of the people that are interested to be part of a group like this, just drop me a message on my Facebook page:
www.facebook.com/ruxandrateach

You Reached Your Slimness Goal Now What?

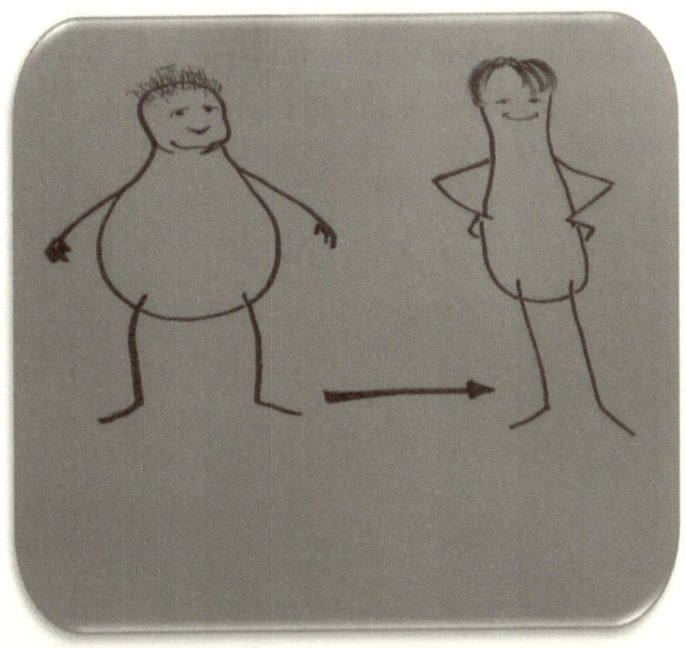

When you've reached your slim, fit, trim goal, and you wonder what to do now, it is very simple. Little by little you increase your calorie intake each day. But make sure that the calorie intake is not more than the calories burned each day, because if it's more, you will gain weight again.

By the time you reach your goal, you will already know roughly how many calories are on your plate. You'll be used to making better decisions, and you'll be able to control the portion sizes. So, from this point on, just maintain control, and keep in mind how much you are eating and burning all day. And that's it. It's easy as that, and you can keep it up for life. On days you exercise, you eat more. On sedentary days, you eat less. By now, you will know all the tricks, and you will know yourself and your body better.

I wish you good luck and all the best in your journey!

THE END

About the Author

Ruxandra Ana Maria Dzubaila is a popular motivational speaker and life coach, specializing in helping people overcome challenges. She focuses her own brand of powerful, life-changing energy on issues like depression, addictions, weight loss, and relationship problems, not to mention helping people manage career transitions and build businesses.

She has traveled extensively throughout Europe and has spent much time both teaching and learning in India and the Far East. With plans to conquer the world with her unique message of hope and transformation, Ruxandra will likely be coming to a city near you before long.

The driving force of Ruxandra's life right now is connecting with people. She brings deep knowledge of multiple spiritual and psychological traditions, along with an unbridled positive attitude and belief in the goodness and beauty of the universe—and the healing power of self-love.

Connect with Ruxandra

Connect with her on Facebook:
http://www.facebook.com/ruxandrateach

&

Follow her on Twitter: @ruxandrateach

Resources

The conclusions outlined in this book are the result of reading many books and doing much research over the course of several of years. Unfortunately, I can't remember them all so I can't list them all here. Instead, the list below contains some of the most important books that I have found, which have played an important role in changing my life and helping me learn the things I needed to know in order to bring this book to life. I highly recommend that you read them. They had a positive impact on my life, and I'm positive they will benefit you just as much.

1. *Awaken the Giant Within* – Tony Robbins
2. *Unlimited Power* – Tony Robbins
3. *The Silva Mind Control Method* – Jose Silva
4. *Unlimited* – Jillian Michaels
5. *The Seven Spiritual Laws of Success* – Deepak Chopra
6. *What Are You Hungry For?* – Deepak Chopra
7. *The Monk Who Sold His Ferrari* – Robin Sharma
8. *Fat to Fearless* – Asher Fox

9. *The New Encyclopedia of Modern Bodybuilding* – Arnold Schwarzenegger
10. *Personal Trainer Manual* – American Council of Exercise
11. *Psycho Cybernetics* – Maxwell Maltz
12. *As a Man Thinketh* – James Allen
13. *You Can Heal Your Life* - Louise Hay
14. *Heal Your Body* – Louise Hay
15. *The Power Is Within You* – Loose Hay
16. *I Can See Clearly Now* – Dr. Wayne Dyer
17. *Dying to Be Me* – Anita Moorjani
18. *Maximize Your Potential Through the Power of Your Subconscious Mind* – Dr. Joseph Murphy
19. *The Power of Your Subconscious Mind* – Dr. Joseph Murphy
20. *The Biology of Belief* – Bruce Lipton
21. *Jillian Michaels Show* – Podcast on iTunes

www.ingramcontent.com/pod-product-compliance
Lightning Source LLC
Chambersburg PA
CBHW050416290526
45786CB00003B/1288